USING

VALERIAN ROOT

FOR BEGINNERS

Unlocking Natural Wellness For Enhanced Well-Being, Reduce Anxiety, Boost Overall Health And More

DR. SPARKS RUBIO

DISCLAIMER

The information presented in this book is intended for general informational purposes only. It is not a substitute for professional medical advice, diagnosis, or treatment.

The author and publisher of this book have made every effort to ensure that the information provided is accurate and up-to-date at the time of publication. However, medical and scientific knowledge is constantly evolving, and new research may emerge. Therefore, the information in this book should not be considered a definitive source for medical or nutritional advice.

It is essential to consult with a qualified healthcare professional before making any decisions.

The author and publisher disclaim any liability for any adverse outcomes or consequences resulting from the use or misuse of the information in this book. Readers are urged to use their discretion and judgment when making decisions about their health and wellness.

By reading this book, you agree to do so at your own risk and should not use it as a substitute for professional medical advice or treatment.

TABLE OF CONTENTS

CHAPTER ONE

INTRODUCTION TO VALERIAN ROOT

ORIGINS AND HISTORY

The herbaceous perennial plant Valeriana officinalis, scientifically known as "valerian root," is indigenous to Europe and some regions of Asia. Its therapeutic powers have earned it great respect in ancient cultures, which is where its history begins. Since the root of Valerian has sedative and relaxing properties, people have used it since ancient Greece and Rome. It is thought that the Latin word "Valera," which means "to be strong" or "to be healthy," is where the name "Valerian" originated, highlighting the plant's long-standing reputation as a herb that improves health.

KNOWING VALERIAN: IT'S BOTANICAL AND CHEMICAL MAKE-UP

Valerian root is a visually attractive botanical specimen, distinguished by its sturdy, tall stem with clusters of sweet-scented, pink or white flowers. The pharmacological actions of this substance make its chemical composition particularly interesting. A variety of active substances, including volatile oils like isovaleric acid, bornyl acetate, and valeric acid, are present in the root and are assumed to have a role in its calming effects. Furthermore, it is known that valerian root contains flavonoids, alkaloids, and other phytochemicals that work together to influence the plant's medicinal properties.

TRADITIONAL USES OF VALERIAN MEDICINE

Traditional medicine has used Valerian extensively throughout history. It was used to alleviate headaches, uneasiness, and insomnia in ancient Greece. In traditional Chinese medicine, it was used to treat digestive problems and menstrual cramps. Throughout the middle Ages, Valerian root was still widely utilized as a cure for a variety of nerve illnesses. When tension and anxiety levels were very high, its sedative qualities were highly prized. Due to its apparent efficacy in treating a variety of conditions, such as anxiety, stress-related diseases, and sleep difficulties, this herb has been included in many cultural pharmacopeias over the years.

Although Valerian has been used for a very long time, its exact mode of action has not been fully understood until recently.

CHAPTER TWO

THE KNOWLEDGE BEHIND VALERIAN ROOT

VALERIAN'S POTENT INGREDIENTS

Since ancient times, people have utilized Valerian root, formally known as Valeriana officinalis, for its supposed health advantages, especially in easing stress and facilitating sleep. Many active chemicals found in this herb are thought to be the cause of its medicinal benefits. The main bioactive components among them are valerenic acid and its derivatives. The brain's gamma-aminobutyric acid (GABA) receptors, which are known to control neuronal excitability, are impacted by valerenic acid. To a lesser degree, other substances such as alkaloids, flavonoids, and valepotriates also contribute to the pharmacological activity of Valerian.

HOW THE BODY REACTS TO VALERIAN

Examining Valerian's relationship with the GABA system is necessary to comprehend how it functions in the body. Research has demonstrated that valerenic acid can prevent GABA from being broken down in the brain, which raises GABA levels. An inhibitory neurotransmitter that aids in controlling neuronal excitability is

GABA. Valerian has a relaxing impact on the neurological system by increasing GABA activity, which lowers anxiety and promotes relaxation. Although the exact mechanism of Valerian is more complex and unclear, it is similar to those of certain popular anti-anxiety drugs.

INVESTIGATIONS AND CLINICAL RESEARCH

Numerous investigations and clinical trials have examined the effectiveness of Valerian in diverse settings. Many studies have looked into the possibility of using Valerian to treat insomnia, and some of them suggest that it may shorten the time it takes to fall asleep and enhance the quality of sleep. These research findings, however, have been somewhat inconsistent; while some have shown clear advantages, others have had more subtle effects. Variations in study designs, dosages, and the populations being studied may be the cause of the inconsistent results. Furthermore, studies on the anxiolytic properties of Valerian have yielded encouraging findings, indicating the herb's potential as a natural substitute for prescription anti-anxiety drugs.

To further understand the safety profile of Valerian, more research has been done. When taken for brief periods and in the recommended dosages, it is generally regarded as safe. On the other hand, excessive dosages or extended use may cause adverse effects such as headaches, nausea, and dizziness. Caution is also warranted due to potential interactions with other drugs.

The current corpus of research suggests that Valerian may have potential as a natural treatment for several anxiety and sleep-related disorders, even if more thorough clinical trials are required to clarify the entire range of Valerian's benefits and its long-term safety. Before adding Valerian to any wellness program, people should, however, speak with a healthcare provider, especially if they have any underlying medical concerns or are taking any medications that may interfere with it.

CHAPTER THREE

USING VALERIAN ROOT AS A NATURAL ADEQUACY

VALERIAN ROOT FOR INSOMNIA AND SLEEP

Because of its possible sedative and anxiolytic effects, Valerian root, which is produced from the Valeriana officinalis plant, has been used for millennia as a natural cure for a variety of health issues. Managing sleep disorders and insomnia is one of the most prominent uses of valerian root. Valerian has been used as an herbal supplement to help those who struggle with sleep disruptions relax and get better quality sleep. It is thought to work with the brain's GABA receptors, which are connected to the control of anxiety and sleep. Valerian may have a sedative effect that speeds up the process of falling asleep and promotes deeper, more restful sleep by making more GABA available.

LOWERING STRESS AND ANXIETY

Moreover, studies have indicated that Valerian root may help lower tension and anxiety levels. Around the world, anxiety disorders are a common mental health problem, and many people look for non-pharmacological ways to treat their symptoms. It is believed that Valerian's ability to reduce anxiety is related to how it affects the release and absorption of neurotransmitters like serotonin. Valerian may assist in regulating mood and lessen jitteriness or uneasiness by adjusting the amounts of these neurotransmitters. Researchers and practitioners alike are nevertheless interested in Valerian because of its historical usage as an anxiolytic drug, even if further clinical trials are needed to determine the particular mechanisms at work.

Furthermore, Valerian root has demonstrated potential in the treatment of panic disorders, which are typified by unexpected, recurrent panic episodes and a continual worry of having further attacks. Even though the precise cause of panic disorders is unknown and complicated, valerian has become more popular as a supplemental treatment because of its possible calming properties. It is thought that valerian may help control the elevated physiological reactions linked to panic attacks by interacting with neurotransmitters like serotonin and

GABA. Valerian root should, however, be taken into account as a component of a thorough treatment plan. People who suffer from severe anxiety or panic disorders should speak with medical professionals for a suitable and all-encompassing method of controlling their illness.

Valerian root has made a name for itself in the field of natural sedatives and anxiolytics, providing a possible substitute for those who favor non-pharmacological interventions or look for complementary therapies to support traditional medical treatments. Its potential as an herbal treatment is supported by its historical use and increasing body of research; nonetheless, more thorough clinical trials are required to completely understand its mechanisms and maximize its use in clinical practice. To guarantee the proper and safe usage of Valerian root, as with any herbal supplement, it is imperative to use caution and speak with a healthcare expert, especially when suffering from persistent sleep difficulties, anxiety, or panic disorders.

CHAPTER FOUR

BENEFITS OF VALERIAN FOR HEALTH

Native to Europe and Asia, valerian is a perennial herb that has been used for its many health advantages. These include possible effects on high blood pressure, pain relief, and gastrointestinal health. While investigations into the exact mechanisms are still underway, certain studies have shed light on how it affects these particular facets of human health.

VITALDIANT AND HYPERTENSION

According to some early studies, valerian may have a moderate hypotensive impact on high blood pressure, which could help lower blood pressure levels. Some of the components included in valerian are thought to have a relaxing impact on the nervous system, which may cause vasodilation and lower blood pressure in general. More thorough research is necessary to determine the exact dosage and long-term consequences for hypertensive patients, though.

Regarding its analgesic effects, valerian has shown encouraging results in the field of pain management. Some components of valerian root have shown promise in reducing pain, possibly through modulating the neurotransmitters linked to pain perception. Valerian's natural characteristics make it a tempting option for people looking for complementary or alternative techniques to managing mild to moderate pain, even though it might not be as effective as some pharmaceutical pain medications.

VALERIAN FOR THE DIGESTIVE SYSTEM

Valerian has demonstrated promise in treating specific gastrointestinal problems when it comes to digestive health. Its anti-spasmodic and muscle-relaxant qualities may aid in easing the symptoms of illnesses including dyspepsia and irritable bowel syndrome (IBS). Additionally, as stress is known to exacerbate several digestive problems, valerian may indirectly improve gastrointestinal health by encouraging relaxation and lowering stress levels.

While valerian shows promise in these areas, it's crucial to remember that each person's reaction to its effects will be different. It is also important to take into account any possible negative effects and how it may mix with specific medications. Although valerian is widely thought to be safe for short-term usage, further research is needed to determine its long-term effects and ideal dosages.

Valerian offers itself as a helpful natural therapy with the ability to improve gastrointestinal health, pain management, and high blood pressure. Before adding valerian to their treatment regimens, people should always speak with medical specialists, especially if they have any underlying medical concerns or are taking any medications that may interfere with this plant. Careful thought should be given to incorporating valerian into holistic wellness techniques, with a focus on the need for thorough study and individualized advice from medical professionals.

VALERIAN IN CONTEMPORARY HEALTH

Because of its potential health benefits, the perennial flowering plant known as valerian, which is native to Europe and parts of Asia, has attracted a lot of attention in the field of modern medicine. Its alleged therapeutic benefits on anxiety and sleep disorders have driven most of its use in pharmaceutical goods. To offer natural substitutes for synthetic sedatives and anxiolytics, extracts from the root of the Valerian plant, which are well-known for their sedative qualities, have been added to several pharmaceutical formulations, such as tinctures, pills, and capsules.

Many nations have strict regulatory monitoring over the use of valerian in pharmaceutical goods due to safety concerns and regulatory constraints. Comprehensive preclinical and clinical investigations are usually necessary for health authorities to evaluate the quality, safety, and efficacy of any valerian-containing product. To guarantee the purity and consistency of the active ingredients in these medicines, compliance with additional quality requirements and Good Manufacturing Practices (GMP) is essential. To guarantee the safe use of medications containing valerian, regulatory agencies frequently require full labeling that includes pertinent cautions, contraindications, and potential bad effects.

It is important to consider the possible interactions and negative effects of valerian despite its generally positive safety profile. Its use is frequently accompanied by modest gastrointestinal disturbances, such as nausea and discomfort in the abdomen. People may occasionally get headaches, lightheadedness, or paradoxical excitability. Long-term use or large dosages of valerian may cause side effects like tiredness and sluggishness during the day. Furthermore, some people may experience adverse reactions when exposed to valerian, so it's important to watch closely and consider alternate treatments.

Additionally, valerian may interact with other drugs and substances, which could be dangerous for people with particular medical conditions. Due to its sedative qualities, using valerian at the same time as other CNS depressants, such as alcohol or some prescription sedatives, might amplify the sedative effects, impairing cognition or causing excessive sleepiness. Moreover, valerian may interfere with the metabolism of pharmaceuticals that are processed by particular liver enzymes, changing their toxicity profiles or efficacy. Therefore, people taking these medications should exercise caution.

CHAPTER FIVE

TYPES AND STRENGTHS OF VALERIAN

SUPPLEMENTS WITH VALERIAN

Native to Europe and Asia, valerian is a perennial herb well known for its possible medical benefits, especially for easing anxiety and insomnia symptoms and promoting relaxation. Supplements containing valerian root are often used as herbal treatments for insomnia and anxiety. Because of its active ingredients, which include valerenic acid and valepotriates, valerian is known for its calming effects. It can be found in many forms, the most popular being tinctures and teas.

BLENDS AND HERBAL TEAS

The process of soaking Valerian root in a solution of alcohol and water yields tinctures, a concentrated liquid form of Valerian extract. The medicinal ingredients in the herb can be extracted using this method, yielding a powerful remedy. Tinctures are preferred because of how convenient they are and how long their shelf life is. Usually, a few drops are diluted with water or another beverage before consumption. Consumers value its rapid absorption because, in comparison to other forms, it can cause effects to manifest sooner.

In contrast, the process of making Valerian teas entails steeping dried Valerian root in hot water to extract its active ingredients. Many people prefer this infusion method as a gentler alternative to tinctures because it has a milder effect and is less concentrated. Due to its well-known calming qualities, Valerian tea is a favorite among people looking to establish a peaceful nighttime routine. Its easy preparation and delicious flavor make it popular among people looking for natural ways to enhance the quality of their sleep.

APPROPRIATE ADMINISTRATION AND DOSAGES

To achieve the intended results and prevent any negative responses, it is essential to determine the appropriate quantities and methods of administering Valerian supplements. While dosage recommendations can change based on variables like age, weight, and particular medical problems, it is generally advised that adults take 300–600 mg of valerenic acid-standardized Valerian extract, which is standardized to contain 0.8% valerenic acid, 30–2 hours before bed.

The usual suggested dosage for tinctures is between 0.5 and 2 milliliters, taken up to three times daily. It is crucial to adhere to the directions on the product label and get individual dosing advice from a medical practitioner. In a similar vein, one to two grams of dried Valerian root should be steeped in a cup of hot water for ten to fifteen minutes, up to three times a day, depending on tolerance and reaction.

Individual reactions to Valerian supplements may differ, so it's best to start with a lower dosage, monitor your tolerance, and modify as necessary. Furthermore, since Valerian may interact with several medications, including sedatives, anti-seizure drugs, and anesthetics, it is imperative to speak with a healthcare professional, particularly when considering long-term use or combining Valerian with other prescriptions. It's critical to understand the proper dosage and method of taking Valerian supplements to guarantee their safe and efficient application in enhancing relaxation and improving the quality of sleep.

CHAPTER SIX

SELECTING HIGH-QUALITY VALERIAN ITEMS

OBTAINING AND EXPANDING VALERIAN

Valerian requires knowledge of the ideal growing conditions to be sourced and grown. Native to Europe and parts of Asia, Valerian is a perennial flowering plant that does best in moist, well-drained soil that receives some shade. Care must be taken during cultivation to guarantee that the soil is sufficiently fertile and has a pH of 5.5 to 7.0. Since organic farming methods don't use artificial fertilizers or pesticides, the final product is typically purer. This makes organic farming practices popular. Sustainable harvesting methods are also necessary to stop depletion and protect the plant's natural habitat.

METHODS OF PROCESSING AND EXTRACTION

The techniques used for extraction and processing have a big influence on the quality of valerian products. Since the roots of the Valerian plant have the largest concentration of the active ingredients that give the plant its therapeutic properties, these parts are usually used in the extraction process. To maintain their bioactive components, the roots are often picked, carefully cleaned, and then dried at regulated temperatures. To create strong and concentrated Valerian extracts, the extraction procedure frequently uses methods like solvent extraction or steam distillation. To guarantee that the finished product maintains its optimum potency and purity, it is essential to maintain the right temperature, pressure, and extraction duration.

HOW TO RECOGNIZE REAL VALERIAN PRODUCTS

Knowing the telltale signs that separate real products from fake or subpar substitutes is essential to recognizing real Valerian products.

First and foremost, you must confirm where the Valerian is coming from and make sure it comes from respectable organic farms with certification or sustainable wildcrafting methods. Furthermore, real products are frequently put through stringent quality testing to ensure that no impurities, heavy metals, or dangerous compounds are present. Transparent labeling is a critical indicator of a product's legitimacy and quality. It includes information about the plant's origins, extraction techniques, and established quantities of essential active ingredients. The product's legitimacy is further confirmed by third-party certifications and regulatory body endorsements, which guarantee that it conforms with industry standards and safety laws.

When it comes to Valerian products, customers ought to give preference to companies that value openness and maintain strict quality control procedures through manufacturing. This entails following industry standards for herbal supplements and utilizing Good Manufacturing Practices (GMP). Testing for purity, potency, and the presence of contaminants in batches is one of the most important quality assurance procedures used to confirm the legitimacy of Valerian products. Furthermore, buying from reputable manufacturers, wholesalers, or merchants who have a reputation for providing high-quality herbal supplements can greatly reduce the chance of buying phony or subpar items. When selecting genuine Valerian products, regular consultation with informed specialists in the field of herbal medicine can also yield insightful advice.

CHAPTER SEVEN

INCLUDING VALERIAN IN YOUR DAILY ROUTINE FOR WELLNESS

VALERIAN IN COMBINATION WITH OTHER HERBS

Due to its relaxing and calming qualities, Valerian makes a powerful and all-encompassing combination when blended with other herbs. One popular combination is Valerian with chamomile, a herb known for its calming properties. Combining these two herbs can result in a potent mixture that helps reduce tension and anxiety while encouraging relaxation. Valerian's calming effects can also be enhanced when combined with passionflower, which promotes deeper feelings of calm and better-quality sleep. These herbs work best together to create a more complete and effective relaxing cure.

USING VALERIAN IN FRAGRANCES

Valerian's unique and unmistakable earthy scent is helping it establish a greater and greater role in the field of aromatherapy. Valerian can help produce a relaxing and peaceful atmosphere when used as an essential oil, which is great for lowering stress and encouraging relaxation. Its scent is frequently characterized as musky, warm, and grounded, which makes it a great option for aromatherapy blends intended to ease anxiety and improve sleep. Valerian essential oil, when diffused, can assist in establishing an environment that is favorable to profound relaxation, enabling people to decompress and settle into a peaceful mood.

VALERIAN COOKING WITH HIM

Valerian is not as frequently used in cooking as other herbs, but it can still be creatively incorporated into a variety of culinary projects. Some dishes go well with its rich, earthy flavor profile, especially those with bold, complimentary notes. Valerian, when used sparingly, can provide savory meals like stews and soups with a distinct and delicate note, adding an aromatic depth that balances the flavor profile overall. Valerian can also be infused into some drinks, giving teas and some cocktails a unique herbal undertone. Its strong flavor should be carefully considered because, if not used sparingly, it can quickly overshadow the dish.

CHAPTER EIGHT

WARNING SIGNS AND EXCLUSIONS

PREGNANCY AND VALERIAN

Due to its possible sedative and anxiolytic properties, the plant valerian, which is native to Europe and some regions of Asia, is frequently taken as a dietary supplement. Its alleged benefits in reducing anxiety and enhancing sleep quality have made it more well-liked, but using it while pregnant is extremely risky and closely monitored. Though it has been historically used to treat several ailments, including sleeplessness, there isn't much scientific data to back up its safety during pregnancy. Because there isn't much thorough research on how it affects expectant mothers and their fetuses, medical professionals frequently recommend against consuming it during this critical time. To protect the health of the developing fetus and the mother, pregnant women should speak with their healthcare practitioners before taking any kind of herbal supplement, including valerian.

When taking certain medications with valerian, there is a chance of drug interactions, thus people should be informed of the potential repercussions of doing so. Because of its well-known sedative qualities, Valerian may interact with other medications that have comparable effects, enhancing the sedative effect overall and increasing feelings of sleepiness or vertigo. These kinds of interactions can be dangerous, particularly for people who are running heavy machinery or performing other tasks that need a high level of awareness. Furthermore, mixing valerian with CNS depressants like alcohol, antihistamines, or benzodiazepines may intensify the sedative effects and increase the likelihood of negative side effects.

Furthermore, concomitant usage of valerian and other drugs, such as anticonvulsants, may lessen the effectiveness of the former, resulting in less-than-ideal therapeutic results. Therefore, before adding valerian to a daily routine, people with underlying health conditions—especially those who are already receiving treatment with specific medications—should proceed with caution and see a medical practitioner. Although valerian is usually considered a safe herb when used as directed, it is important to consult a healthcare provider before beginning any new supplementation regimen that includes valerian due to the possibility of drug interactions.

Moreover, it is important to consider the possibility of negative interactions between valerian and other drugs. When valerian is used alongside other sedative-containing plants or supplements, like kava or St. John's wort, the sedative effects may intensify, possibly causing extreme tiredness and a reduction in cognitive function.

CONCLUSION

CONSERVATION AND SUSTAINABILITY

The importance of sustainability and conservation in global discourse has increased as awareness of the effects of human activity on the environment has grown. The pressing need to implement sustainable practices has increased in the last several years due to the startling rates of depletion of natural resources and the worsening of climate change. The idea of satisfying current demands without sacrificing the capacity of future generations to satisfy their wants is included in the concept of sustainability. In this setting, there has been an increase in interest in sustainable development across several industries, such as manufacturing, agriculture, and energy. It entails finding a careful balance between social progress, environmental preservation, and economic growth. Many countries and organizations now place a high priority on preserving biodiversity, using renewable energy sources, reducing waste, and practicing responsible consumption.

Furthermore, the preservation of the Earth's unique species and fragile ecosystems has made conservation activities increasingly important. To guarantee the sustainable use of natural resources for future generations, conservation entails their management and protection. This frequently means creating protected areas, putting policies in place to preserve animals, and controlling human activity that can endanger the environment. Conservation activities are essential to preserving ecological balance, reducing the loss of important ecosystems, and averting the extinction of fragile species, in addition to protecting biodiversity. Conservation efforts serve a critical role in promoting a more harmonious connection between humans and the planet by deepening our understanding of the interconnectedness between human actions and the natural world.

TRENDS IN THE USE OF VALERIAN

Turning our attention to the use of Valerian, we can see that there has been a noticeable upsurge in the popularity of this herbal medicine in the health and wellness sector. Known for its sedative and anxiolytic qualities, Valerian root has long been used to treat a wide range of conditions, such as anxiety and insomnia. The potential advantages of Valerian root in fostering relaxation and enhancing the quality of sleep have come to light more and more recently. This has raised consumer demand for items containing valerian, such as teas, pills, and essential oils, which are sold to those looking for all-natural cures for stress and sleep issues. Furthermore, the incorporation of Valerian into complementary and alternative medicine methods has facilitated the herb's broad recognition as a comprehensive strategy for treating specific physiological and psychological ailments.

DIFFICULTIES

But even with all of this interest in Valerian, there are still several issues that need to be addressed. Regulating

Valerian-based goods to ensure their safety, effectiveness, and uniform quality is one of the main concerns. Some areas may have lax regulatory regimes that encourage the production of inferior goods, endangering the health of consumers and undermining the validity of Valerian as a trustworthy natural treatment. To avoid overexploitation and the destruction of the plant's natural habitats, it is also necessary to carefully control the sustainability of the cultivation and harvesting methods for Valerian. Maintaining the long-term availability and ecological integrity of Valerian will require striking a balance between the growing demand for the plant and ethical sourcing methods. To address these issues and ensure consumer safety, as well as environmental preservation, industry stakeholders, regulatory bodies, and environmental experts, must work together to establish comprehensive guidelines for the sustainable cultivation, manufacturing, and distribution of Valerian products.

www.ingramcontent.com/pod-product-compliance
Lightning Source LLC
Chambersburg PA
CBHW060806260726
48660CB00002B/812